COLITIS DIET COOKBOOK FOR SENIORS OVER 50

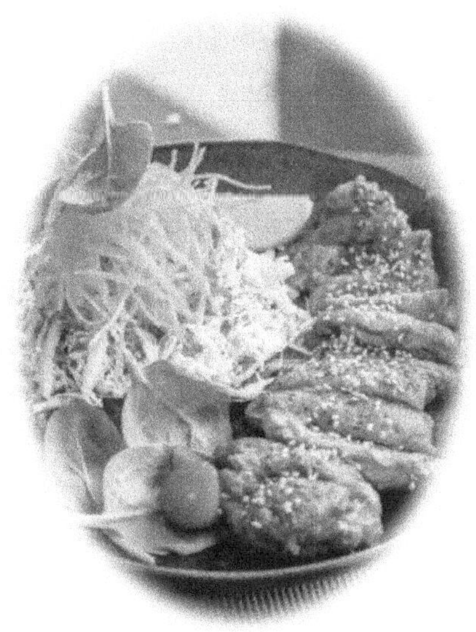

Culinary Care: Nourishing Solutions for
Seniors Overcoming Colitis with Flavorful

Dr. Fawn Henry

Copyright © [2024] by [Dr. Fawn Henry**]**

Reserved all rights. This publication cannot be duplicated, shared, or transmitted in any way without the publisher's prior written consent. The only exceptions are brief quotes used in critical evaluations and certain other noncommercial uses allowed by copyright law. Such uses include photocopying, recording, and other electronic or mechanical methods

TABLE OF CONTENTS

CONCLUSION 91

INTRODUCTION

Welcome to the "Colitis Diet Cookbook for Seniors Over 50: Delicious and Nutritious Low-Carb and Low-Sugar Recipes for Elders." I'm Dr. Fawn Henry, a nutritionist with years of experience helping people harness the power of nutrition to manage their health. This cookbook is a labor of love, inspired by my passion for food and my commitment to improving the lives of those living with colitis.

Living with colitis can be incredibly challenging, especially for seniors who may already be dealing with a host of other health issues. The discomfort, pain, and dietary restrictions can make everyday meals a daunting task. However, I firmly believe that the right nutrition can make a significant difference, not just in managing symptoms, but in enhancing overall well-being. This cookbook aims to provide you with a collection of recipes that are not only suitable for managing colitis but also delicious and satisfying.

Allow me to share a story that is particularly close to my heart. My dear friend Jessica, who is in her early 60s, was diagnosed with colitis a few years ago. Jessica is a vibrant, active woman who loves gardening, painting, and spending time with her grandchildren. However, her diagnosis left her feeling overwhelmed and frustrated. She struggled with constant abdominal pain, unpredictable flare-ups, and a lack of energy, which significantly impacted her quality of life.

Jessica tried various medications and treatments, but the relief was temporary and came with unwanted side effects. Watching her suffer, I knew I had to step in and help her find a more sustainable solution. I started by analyzing her diet, identifying foods that triggered her symptoms, and those that could potentially soothe her inflamed digestive tract.

Together, we embarked on a journey of nutritional discovery. We focused on anti-inflammatory foods, rich in nutrients and easy to digest. We incorporated more lean proteins, healthy fats, and low-carb vegetables into her diet while cutting down on sugar and processed foods. I introduced her to the wonders of gut-healing broths, fiber-rich seeds, and the importance of hydration.

One of the turning points for Jessica was when she realized that eating well didn't mean giving up on taste or pleasure. We experimented with herbs and spices to add flavor without causing irritation. We created meal plans that were simple, yet packed with nutrients. Jessica started to notice a difference within weeks. Her energy levels improved, her flare-ups became less frequent, and she began to enjoy her meals again.

Jessica's journey was a testament to the incredible impact of nutrition. Her transformation inspired me to create this cookbook, to share the same principles and recipes that helped her regain control over her health.

Each recipe in this book has been carefully crafted to ensure it's not only beneficial for managing colitis but also enjoyable to eat.

What You'll Find in This Cookbook

This cookbook is designed with seniors in mind. The recipes are straightforward, easy to prepare, and focus on ingredients that are gentle on the digestive system. You'll find a variety of meals, from hearty breakfasts and refreshing salads to comforting soups and satisfying dinners. Each recipe is low in carbs and sugar, helping to reduce inflammation and support gut health.

I hope that this cookbook becomes a valuable resource in your kitchen, providing you with the tools and inspiration to manage colitis through the power of nutrition. Here's to delicious meals and better health!

CHAPTER 1

Colitis, a term used to describe inflammation of the colon (large intestine), can cause a range of symptoms that significantly impact a person's quality of life. To manage colitis effectively, it's crucial to understand its various types, underlying causes, common symptoms, and preventive measures. This comprehensive guide aims to provide a thorough understanding of colitis, helping those affected by the condition to make informed decisions about their health.

Types of Colitis

Colitis can be classified into several types, each with distinct causes and characteristics:

1. **Ulcerative Colitis (UC):** Ulcerative colitis is a chronic inflammatory bowel disease (IBD) that causes long-lasting inflammation and ulcers in the innermost lining of the colon and rectum.

It typically begins in the rectum and can extend to other parts of the colon.

2. **Crohn's Disease**: Although Crohn's disease can affect any part of the gastrointestinal tract, it is included here because it often involves the colon. Crohn's disease causes inflammation that can penetrate deeper layers of the intestinal wall, unlike the superficial inflammation seen in UC.

3. **Microscopic Colitis**: This type of colitis is characterized by inflammation that is only visible under a microscope. It includes two subtypes:

   - **Collagenous Colitis**: Marked by a thick layer of collagen under the lining of the colon.

   - **Lymphocytic Colitis**: Characterized by an increased number of lymphocytes (a type of white blood cell) in the colon lining.

4. **Infectious Colitis**: Caused by bacterial, viral, or parasitic infections, this type of colitis results from pathogens such as Salmonella, Shigella, and Campylobacter. These infections lead to inflammation and can be acute or chronic.

5. **Ischemic Colitis**: Ischemic colitis occurs when blood flow to part of the colon is reduced, often due to narrowed or blocked arteries. This reduction in blood flow can cause pain and damage to the colon.

6. **Radiation Colitis**: Radiation colitis can develop after radiation therapy for cancer, particularly when the abdomen or pelvis is targeted. The radiation can damage the lining of the colon, leading to inflammation.

7. **Drug-Induced Colitis**: Certain medications, such as nonsteroidal anti-inflammatory drugs (NSAIDs), antibiotics, and chemotherapy agents, can cause colitis as a side effect.

Causes of Colitis

The causes of colitis vary depending on the type:

1. **Genetic Factors**: Genetics play a significant role, particularly in ulcerative colitis and Crohn's disease. Individuals with a family history of these conditions are at higher risk.

2. **Immune System Dysfunction**: In autoimmune conditions like ulcerative colitis and Crohn's disease, the immune system mistakenly attacks the healthy cells of the colon, causing inflammation.

3. **Infections**: Pathogens such as bacteria, viruses, and parasites can directly infect the colon, leading to infectious colitis.

4. **Reduced Blood Flow**: Ischemic colitis results from reduced blood flow to the colon, often due to atherosclerosis (hardening of the arteries), blood clots, or other circulatory issues.

5. **Radiation Therapy**: Exposure to radiation during cancer treatment can damage the cells lining the colon, causing radiation colitis.

6. **Medications**: Certain medications can irritate the colon or alter its normal function, leading to inflammation. Examples include NSAIDs, antibiotics, and chemotherapy drugs.

7. **Diet and Lifestyle**: While diet alone doesn't cause colitis, certain foods and lifestyle factors can exacerbate symptoms and contribute to flare-ups in people with existing conditions.

Symptoms of Colitis

The symptoms of colitis can vary widely depending on the type and severity of the condition. Common symptoms include:

1. **Abdominal Pain and Cramping**: Pain is often felt in the lower abdomen and can range from mild to severe.

2. **Diarrhea**: Frequent, loose, and sometimes bloody stools are a hallmark of colitis. Diarrhea may be persistent or intermittent.

3. **Rectal Bleeding**: Blood in the stool is common, particularly in ulcerative colitis and Crohn's disease.

4. **Urgency to Defecate**: A sudden and intense need to have a bowel movement, often with difficulty in controlling it.

5. **Fatigue**: Chronic inflammation and the body's response can lead to persistent tiredness and lack of energy.

6. **Weight Loss**: Unintended weight loss can occur due to malabsorption of nutrients, decreased appetite, and increased metabolic demands of the body dealing with inflammation.

7. **Fever**: Infections and severe inflammation can cause fever and other systemic symptoms.

8. **Joint Pain**: Some types of colitis, especially Crohn's disease, are associated with arthritis and other inflammatory conditions.

Preventive Measures for Colitis

While some forms of colitis cannot be entirely prevented, especially those with genetic or autoimmune origins, there are strategies to reduce the risk of flare-ups and manage symptoms effectively:

1. **Dietary Modifications**:

   - **Anti-Inflammatory Diet**: Incorporate foods rich in omega-3 fatty acids (e.g., fish, flaxseeds), antioxidants (e.g., berries, leafy greens), and fiber (e.g., whole grains, legumes). Avoid processed foods, high-sugar foods, and trans fats.

   - **Low-Residue Diet**: In cases of severe symptoms, a low-residue diet that limits fiber intake can reduce the frequency and volume of bowel movements, easing symptoms.

- **Hydration**: Staying well-hydrated helps maintain bowel function and prevents dehydration from diarrhea.

2. **Regular Exercise**: Physical activity helps reduce stress, improve overall health, and support immune function. Aim for at least 30 minutes of moderate exercise most days of the week.

3. **Stress Management**: Stress can exacerbate colitis symptoms. Techniques such as mindfulness, meditation, yoga, and deep-breathing exercises can help manage stress levels.

4. **Medications and Supplements**:

   - **Anti-Inflammatory Drugs**: Medications such as aminosalicylates and corticosteroids can help control inflammation.

   - **Immunosuppressants**: Drugs that suppress the immune system may be prescribed to prevent immune-mediated inflammation.

- **Probiotics**: These beneficial bacteria can help maintain a healthy gut microbiome, potentially reducing colitis symptoms.

5. **Regular Medical Check-Ups**: Regular visits to a healthcare provider are crucial for monitoring the condition, managing medications, and addressing any new or worsening symptoms promptly.

6. **Avoiding Triggers**: Identify and avoid foods, medications, or activities that trigger symptoms. Keeping a food diary can help pinpoint specific triggers.

7. **Smoking Cessation**: Smoking can worsen symptoms in Crohn's disease, although it has a complex relationship with ulcerative colitis. Quitting smoking is generally beneficial for overall health.

8. **Vaccinations**: Stay up-to-date with vaccinations, as colitis and its treatments can increase susceptibility to infections.

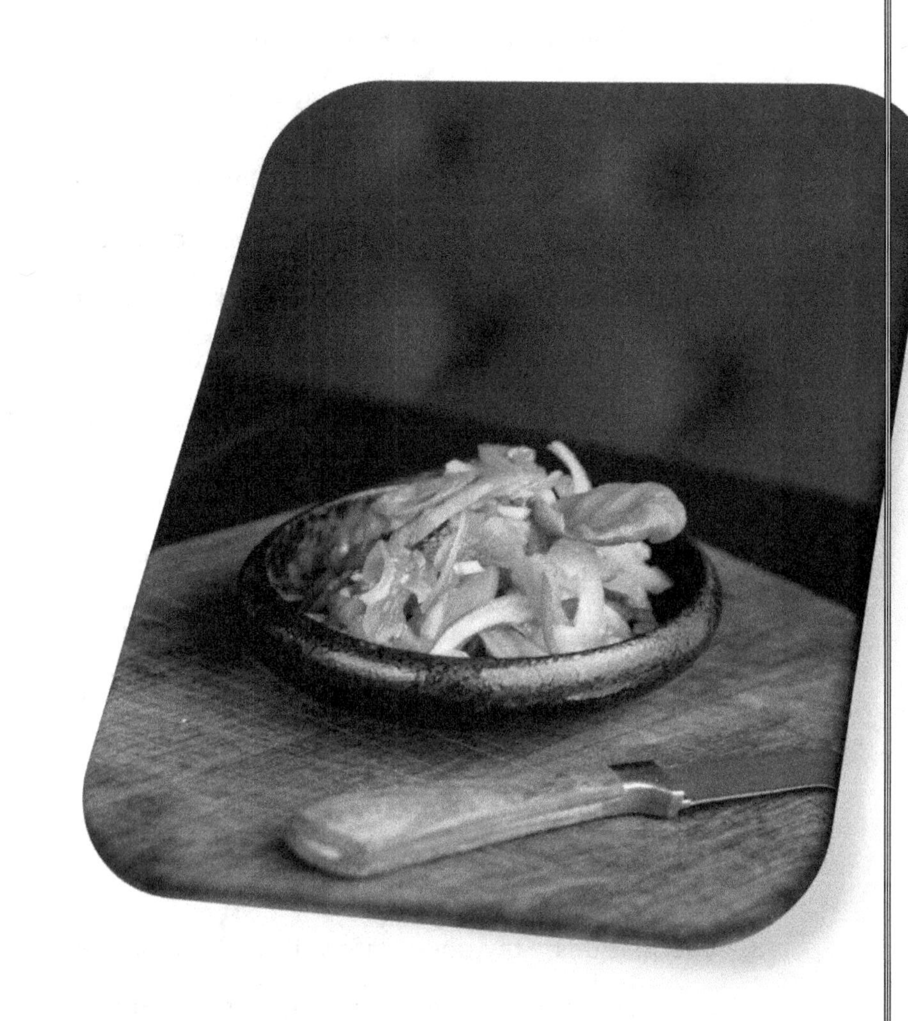

CHAPTER 2

Foods to Eat and Avoid for Optimum Health

Managing colitis through diet is crucial for seniors over 50 to alleviate symptoms, reduce inflammation, and enhance overall health. The right dietary choices can help manage flare-ups, provide necessary nutrients, and improve the quality of life. Here's an in-depth guide to the foods to eat and avoid for seniors with colitis.

Foods to Eat

1. Lean Proteins:

- **Chicken and Turkey**: Skinless poultry is gentle on the digestive system and provides essential proteins without adding excessive fat.

- **Fish**: Fatty fish like salmon, mackerel, and sardines are rich in omega-3 fatty acids, known for their anti-inflammatory properties.

- **Eggs**: Easily digestible and versatile, eggs are a good source of high-quality protein.

2. Low-Fiber Vegetables:

- **Cucumbers, Squash, and Zucchini**: These vegetables are low in fiber and easy to digest, especially when cooked.

- **Carrots and Sweet Potatoes**: Cooking these root vegetables makes them easier to digest while providing essential vitamins and minerals.

3. Fruits Without Skins and Seeds:

- **Bananas**: Soft and easily digestible, bananas are gentle on the gut and provide potassium, which is important for electrolyte balance.

- **Applesauce and Canned Peaches**: These forms of fruit are easier to digest than raw varieties and still offer important nutrients.

4. Refined Grains:

- **White Rice and Pasta**: These are easier on the digestive system compared to whole grains, which can be too fibrous.

- **Oatmeal**: A good source of soluble fiber that is generally well-tolerated and can help soothe the digestive tract.

5. Healthy Fats:

- **Olive Oil and Avocado**: These provide essential fatty acids and have anti-inflammatory properties. Olive oil can be used for cooking, and avocado can be added to salads or smoothies.

- **Nuts and Seeds**: Almonds, chia seeds, and flaxseeds are good sources of healthy fats and fiber. However, they should be consumed in moderation and preferably ground to aid digestion.

6. Low-Lactose Dairy:

- **Yogurt and Kefir**: These fermented dairy products contain probiotics that support gut health. Opt for low-lactose or lactose-free options to avoid digestive discomfort.

- **Lactose-Free Milk**: This can be a good alternative for those who are lactose intolerant but still want to include milk in their diet.

7. Broths and Soups:

- **Bone Broth**: Rich in nutrients and collagen, bone broth can help soothe the gut lining and provide easy-to-digest nourishment.

- **Vegetable Soups**: Made with low-fiber vegetables, these soups can be both nutritious and comforting. Avoid adding heavy creams or spices.

Foods to Avoid

1. High-Fiber Foods:

- **Raw Vegetables and Fruits**: These can be difficult to digest and may irritate the colon. Examples include broccoli, cauliflower, and raw apples.

- **Whole Grains**: Foods like brown rice, whole wheat bread, and quinoa contain too much fiber, which can aggravate symptoms.

2. Spicy and Fried Foods:

- **Hot Peppers and Spicy Sauces**: Spices can exacerbate inflammation and cause discomfort in the digestive tract.

- **Fried Foods**: High in unhealthy fats, fried foods can irritate the colon and worsen symptoms.

3. Dairy Products:

- **Milk and Cheese**: High-lactose dairy products can be difficult to digest and may lead to bloating, gas, and diarrhea.

- **Cream and Butter**: These high-fat dairy products can also irritate the digestive system.

4. High-Fat Meats:

- **Red Meat and Processed Meats**: These are harder to digest and can increase inflammation. Processed meats like sausages and bacon are particularly problematic due to added preservatives and high fat content.

5. Caffeinated and Carbonated Beverages:

- **Coffee and Soda**: These can irritate the gut lining, contribute to dehydration, and exacerbate colitis symptoms.

- **Alcohol**: Alcohol can increase inflammation and interfere with the effectiveness of medications used to treat colitis.

6. Artificial Sweeteners and Additives:

- **Sugar Alcohols (e.g., sorbitol, mannitol)**: Found in sugar-free products, these can cause bloating and diarrhea.

- **Preservatives and Artificial Colors**: These additives can trigger symptoms in sensitive individuals and should be avoided.

7. High-Sugar Foods:

- **Sweets and Pastries**: High-sugar foods can lead to increased inflammation and digestive discomfort.

- **Sugary Beverages**: Soft drinks, fruit punches, and other sugary drinks can exacerbate symptoms.

Tips for Optimal Health

1. Stay Hydrated:

- Drink plenty of water throughout the day. Proper hydration helps maintain bowel function and prevent dehydration, which is particularly important for those experiencing diarrhea.

2. Eat Small, Frequent Meals:

- Smaller, more frequent meals are easier on the digestive system and can help prevent flare-ups. Aim for five to six small meals rather than three large ones.

3. Cook Foods Thoroughly:

- Cooking breaks down fibers and makes foods easier to digest. Steaming, boiling, or baking are preferred methods over frying or grilling.

4. Monitor and Adjust:

- Keeping a food diary can help identify foods that trigger symptoms and those that are well-tolerated. This can be invaluable for making informed dietary choices.

5. Probiotics and Supplements:

- Consider incorporating probiotics to support a healthy gut microbiome. Supplements like omega-3 fatty acids and vitamin D can also support overall health but should be taken under the guidance of a healthcare provider.

6. Manage Stress:

- Stress can exacerbate colitis symptoms. Techniques such as mindfulness, meditation, yoga, and deep-breathing exercises can help manage stress levels.

7. Regular Medical Check-Ups:

- Regular visits to a healthcare provider are crucial for monitoring the condition, managing medications, and addressing any new or worsening symptoms promptly.

8. Avoiding Triggers:

- Identify and avoid foods, medications, or activities that trigger symptoms. This can involve eliminating certain foods from your diet or finding alternatives to medications that cause gastrointestinal distress.

9. Smoking Cessation:

- Smoking can worsen symptoms in Crohn's disease and has a complex relationship with ulcerative colitis. Quitting smoking is generally beneficial for overall health and can improve colitis symptoms.

10. Vaccinations:

- Staying up-to-date with vaccinations is important, as colitis and its treatments can increase susceptibility to infections. Consult with your healthcare provider about appropriate vaccines.

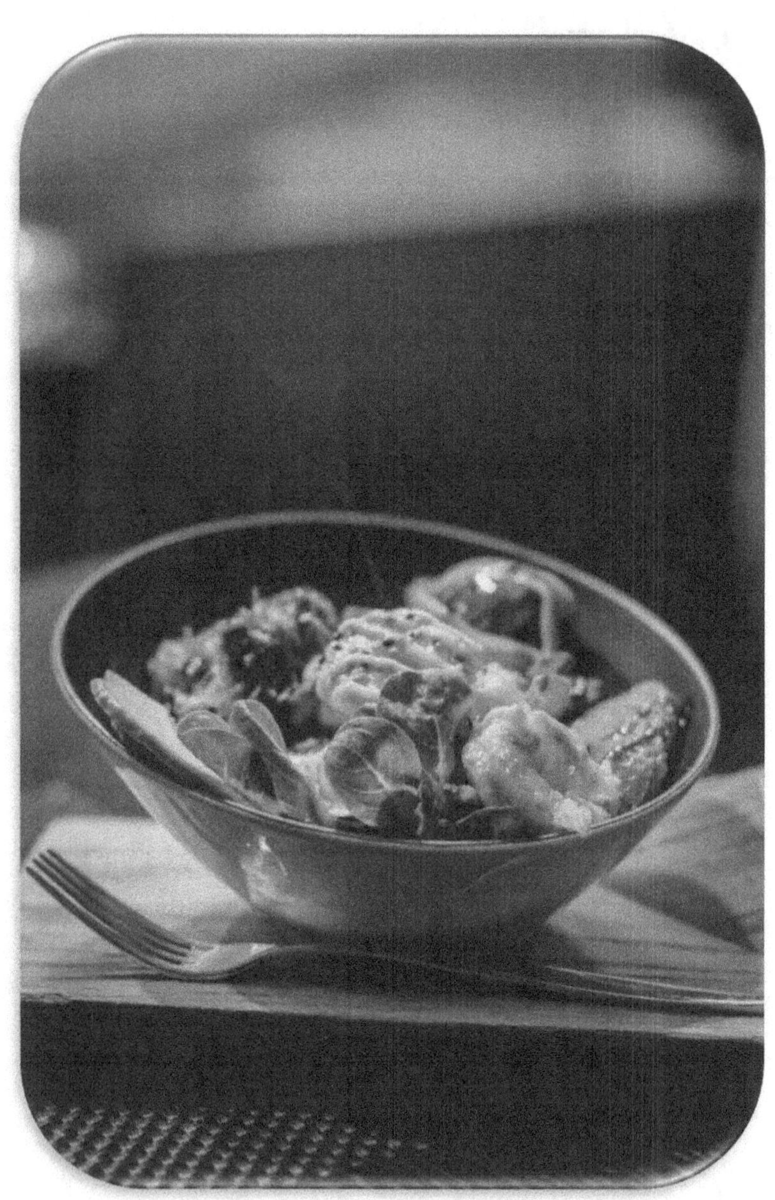

CHAPTER 3

BREAK FAST RECIPES

1. Banana Oatmeal Porridge

Servings: 2

Cooking Time: 10 minutes

Ingredients:

- ❖ 1 cup rolled oats

- ❖ 2 cups water

- ❖ 1 ripe banana, mashed

- ❖ 1/2 teaspoon cinnamon

- ❖ 1 tablespoon chia seeds

- ❖ 1 teaspoon honey (optional)

- ❖ A pinch of salt

Preparation:

1. In a medium saucepan, bring water to a boil.

2. Add oats and a pinch of salt. Reduce heat to low and simmer, stirring occasionally, for about 5 minutes.

3. Stir in the mashed banana, cinnamon, and chia seeds. Cook for another 2 minutes until the oats are tender and creamy.

4. Remove from heat and let sit for a minute to thicken.

5. Serve warm with a drizzle of honey if desired.

Nutritional Value (per serving):

- Calories: 180

- Protein: 5g

- Carbohydrates: 31g

- Fiber: 6g

- Fat: 3g

- Sodium: 40mg

2. Avocado and Spinach Smoothie

Servings: 2

Cooking Time: 5 minutes

Ingredients:

- ❖ 1 ripe avocado

- ❖ 1 cup fresh spinach leaves

- ❖ 1 cup unsweetened almond milk

- ❖ 1/2 cup Greek yogurt (low-fat)

- ❖ 1 tablespoon flaxseed meal

- ❖ 1 teaspoon honey (optional)

Preparation:

1. Cut the avocado in half, remove the pit, and scoop the flesh into a blender.

2. Add the spinach, almond milk, Greek yogurt, and flaxseed meal.

3. Blend on high until smooth and creamy.

4. Taste and add honey if desired. Blend again to combine.

5. Pour into glasses and serve immediately.

Nutritional Value (per serving):

- Calories: 210

- Protein: 8g

- Carbohydrates: 12g

- Fiber: 7g

- Fat: 15g

- Sodium: 80mg

3. Scrambled Eggs with Spinach and Tomato

Servings:2

Cooking Time: 10 minutes

Ingredients:

- ❖ 4 large eggs

- ❖ 1 cup fresh spinach leaves, chopped

- ❖ 1 medium tomato, diced

- ❖ 1 tablespoon olive oil

- ❖ Salt and pepper to taste

Preparation:

1. In a medium bowl, whisk the eggs with a pinch of salt and pepper.

2. Heat olive oil in a non-stick skillet over medium heat.

3. Add the chopped spinach and diced tomato. Cook until the spinach is wilted and the tomato is soft, about 3 minutes.

4. Pour the eggs into the skillet. Stir gently with a spatula until the eggs are fully cooked but still soft, about 3-4 minutes.

5. Serve immediately.

Nutritional Value (per serving):

- Calories: 180

- Protein: 13g

- Carbohydrates: 4g

- Fiber: 2g

- Fat: 13g

- Sodium: 160mg

Servings:2

Cooking Time: 10 minutes (plus 4 hours chilling time)

Ingredients:

- ❖ 1 cup unsweetened almond milk

- ❖ 1/4 cup chia seeds

- ❖ 1/2 cup fresh blueberries

- ❖ 1 teaspoon vanilla extract

- ❖ 1 teaspoon honey (optional)

Preparation:

1. In a medium bowl, whisk together the almond milk, chia seeds, vanilla extract, and honey if using.

2. Stir in the blueberries.

3. Cover and refrigerate for at least 4 hours or overnight, stirring once or twice.

4. Before serving, stir the pudding to ensure even distribution of chia seeds.

5. Serve chilled.

Nutritional Value (per serving):

- Calories: 150

- Protein: 5g

- Carbohydrates: 16g

- Fiber: 10g

- Fat: 7g

- Sodium: 50mg

5. Quinoa Breakfast Bowl

Servings:2

Cooking Time: 15 minutes

Ingredients:

- ❖ 1 cup cooked quinoa

- ❖ 1/2 cup almond milk

- ❖ 1 tablespoon almond butter

- ❖ 1/2 teaspoon cinnamon

- ❖ 1 apple, diced

- ❖ 1 tablespoon pumpkin seeds

Preparation:

1. In a small saucepan, combine the cooked quinoa and almond milk. Heat over medium heat until warm.

2. Stir in the almond butter and cinnamon until well combined.

3. Divide the quinoa mixture between two bowls.

4. Top with diced apple and pumpkin seeds.

5. Serve warm.

Nutritional Value (per serving):

- Calories: 220

- Protein: 7g

- Carbohydrates: 30g

- Fiber: 6g

- Fat: 8g

- Sodium: 60mg

Servings: 2

Cooking Time: 25 minutes

Ingredients:

- ❖ 2 medium apples

- ❖ 1 teaspoon cinnamon

- ❖ 2 tablespoons chopped walnuts

- ❖ 1 teaspoon honey (optional)

Preparation:

1. Preheat the oven to 350°F (175°C).

2. Core the apples and place them in a baking dish.

3. Sprinkle with cinnamon and fill the centers with chopped walnuts.

4. Drizzle with honey if desired.

5. Bake for 20-25 minutes until the apples are tender.

6. Serve warm.

Nutritional Value (per serving):

- Calories: 130

- Protein: 2g

- Carbohydrates: 24g

- Fiber: 5g

- Fat: 5g

- Sodium: 0mg

7. Sweet Potato Hash with Eggs

Servings: 2

Cooking Time: 20 minutes

Ingredients:

- ❖ 1 large sweet potato, peeled and diced

- ❖ 1 small onion, diced

- ❖ 1 red bell pepper, diced

- ❖ 2 tablespoons olive oil

- ❖ 4 large eggs

- ❖ Salt and pepper to taste

Preparation:

1. Heat olive oil in a large skillet over medium heat.

2. Add the diced sweet potato, onion, and bell pepper. Cook, stirring occasionally, until the vegetables are tender, about 10-12 minutes.

3. Make four small wells in the vegetable mixture and crack an egg into each well.

4. Cover the skillet and cook until the eggs are set, about 5 minutes.

5. Season with salt and pepper and serve immediately.

Nutritional Value (per serving):

- Calories: 250

- Protein: 10g

- Carbohydrates: 25g

- Fiber: 4g

- Fat: 13g

- Sodium: 150mg

8. Greek Yogurt with Berries and Honey

Servings:2

Cooking Time: 5 minutes

Ingredients:

- ❖ 1 cup Greek yogurt (low-fat)

- ❖ 1/2 cup mixed berries (blueberries, strawberries, raspberries)

- ❖ 1 teaspoon honey

- ❖ 1 tablespoon chia seeds

Preparation:

1. Divide the Greek yogurt between two bowls.

2. Top each bowl with mixed berries.

3. Drizzle with honey and sprinkle with chia seeds.

4. Serve immediately.

Nutritional Value (per serving):

- Calories: 150

- Protein: 10g

- Carbohydrates: 20g

- Fiber: 5g

- Fat: 3g

- Sodium: 60mg

9. Spinach and Feta Omelette

Servings:2

Cooking Time: 10 minutes

Ingredients:

- ❖ 4 large eggs

- ❖ 1/2 cup fresh spinach, chopped

- ❖ 1/4 cup feta cheese, crumbled

- ❖ 1 tablespoon olive oil

- ❖ Salt and pepper to taste

Preparation:

1. In a medium bowl, whisk the eggs with a pinch of salt and pepper.

2. Heat olive oil in a non-stick skillet over medium heat.

3. Add the spinach and cook until wilted, about 2 minutes.

4. Pour the eggs into the skillet and cook until they begin to set, about 3 minutes.

5. Sprinkle the feta cheese over one half of the omelette.

6. Fold the other half over the cheese and cook for another 2 minutes until the eggs are fully cooked.

7. Serve immediately.

Nutritional Value (per serving):

- Calories: 200

- Protein: 14g

- Carbohydrates: 2g

- Fiber: 1g

- Fat: 15g

- Sodium: 260mg

10. Cottage Cheese with Pineapple and Mint

Servings:2

Cooking Time: 5 minutes

Ingredients:

- ❖ 1 cup low-fat cottage cheese

- ❖ 1/2 cup fresh pineapple, diced

- ❖ 1 tablespoon fresh mint, chopped

Preparation:

1. Divide the cottage cheese between two bowls.

2. Top each bowl with diced pineapple.

3. Sprinkle with fresh mint.

4. Serve immediately.

Nutritional Value (per serving):

- Calories: 120

- Protein: 12g

- Carbohydrates: 12g

- Fiber: 1g

- Fat: 3g

- Sodium: 320mg

CHAPTER 4

LUNCH RECIPES

1. Grilled Chicken and Quinoa Salad

Servings:4

Cooking Time: 30 minutes

Ingredients:

- ❖ 2 cups cooked quinoa

- ❖ 2 grilled chicken breasts, sliced

- ❖ 1 cup cherry tomatoes, halved

- ❖ 1 cucumber, diced

- ❖ 1/4 cup red onion, finely chopped

- ❖ 2 tablespoons olive oil

- ❖ 2 tablespoons lemon juice

- ❖ 1 tablespoon fresh parsley, chopped

- ❖ Salt and pepper to taste

Preparation:

1. Cook the quinoa according to package instructions and let it cool.

2. Grill the chicken breasts until fully cooked, then slice them into thin strips.

3. In a large bowl, combine the quinoa, chicken, cherry tomatoes, cucumber, and red onion.

4. In a small bowl, whisk together the olive oil, lemon juice, parsley, salt, and pepper.

5. Pour the dressing over the salad and toss to combine.

6. Serve chilled or at room temperature.

Nutritional Value (per serving):

- Calories: 250

- Protein: 20g

- Carbohydrates: 22g

- Fiber: 3g

- Fat: 10g

- Sodium: 150mg

2. Vegetable Stir-Fry with Tofu

Servings:4

Cooking Time: 25 minutes

Ingredients:

- ❖ 1 block firm tofu, cubed

- ❖ 1 red bell pepper, sliced

- ❖ 1 yellow bell pepper, sliced

- ❖ 1 zucchini, sliced

- ❖ 1 cup broccoli florets

- ❖ 2 tablespoons olive oil

- ❖ 2 tablespoons low-sodium soy sauce

- ❖ 1 tablespoon ginger, grated

- ❖ 1 garlic clove, minced

- ❖ 1 teaspoon sesame oil (optional)

Preparation:

1. Heat 1 tablespoon of olive oil in a large skillet over medium-high heat.

2. Add the tofu cubes and cook until golden brown on all sides, about 5-7 minutes. Remove from the skillet and set aside.

3. In the same skillet, add the remaining tablespoon of olive oil.

4. Add the ginger and garlic, sautéing for 1 minute until fragrant.

5. Add the bell peppers, zucchini, and broccoli, stirring frequently, and cook for about 5-7 minutes until vegetables are tender.

6. Return the tofu to the skillet and add the soy sauce, stirring to combine.

7. Drizzle with sesame oil if desired and serve immediately.

Nutritional Value (per serving):

- Calories: 180

- Protein: 10g

- Carbohydrates: 12g

- Fiber: 4g

- Fat: 10g

- Sodium: 220mg

3. Turkey Lettuce Wraps

Servings:4

Cooking Time: 20 minutes

Ingredients:

- ❖ 1 lb ground turkey

- ❖ 1/2 cup water chestnuts, chopped

- ❖ 1/2 cup carrots, shredded

- ❖ 1/4 cup green onions, chopped

- ❖ 2 tablespoons low-sodium soy sauce

- ❖ 1 tablespoon hoisin sauce

- ❖ 1 teaspoon ginger, grated

- ❖ 1 garlic clove, minced

- ❖ 1 head of butter lettuce

- ❖ 2 tablespoons olive oil

Preparation:

1. Heat olive oil in a large skillet over medium heat.

2. Add the ground turkey, breaking it apart with a spoon, and cook until browned, about 5-7 minutes.

3. Add the ginger, garlic, water chestnuts, carrots, and green onions, cooking for another 3-4 minutes.

4. Stir in the soy sauce and hoisin sauce, cooking for an additional 2 minutes.

5. Remove from heat and let it cool slightly.

6. Separate the butter lettuce leaves and spoon the turkey mixture into each leaf.

7. Serve immediately.

Nutritional Value (per serving):

- Calories: 200

- Protein: 25g

- Carbohydrates: 8g

- Fiber: 2g

- Fat: 8g

- Sodium: 220mg

4. Quinoa Stuffed Bell Peppers

Servings:4

Cooking Time: 40 minutes

Ingredients:

- ❖ 4 large bell peppers

- ❖ 1 cup cooked quinoa

- ❖ 1 cup black beans, drained and rinsed

- ❖ 1 cup corn kernels

- ❖ 1/2 cup diced tomatoes

- ❖ 1/4 cup chopped cilantro

- ❖ 1 teaspoon cumin

- ❖ 1 teaspoon paprika

- ❖ 2 tablespoons olive oil

- ❖ Salt and pepper to taste

Preparation:

1. Preheat the oven to 375°F (190°C).

2. Cut the tops off the bell peppers and remove the seeds.

3. In a large bowl, combine the quinoa, black beans, corn, tomatoes, cilantro, cumin, paprika, olive oil, salt, and pepper.

4. Stuff each bell pepper with the quinoa mixture and place them in a baking dish.

5. Cover with aluminum foil and bake for 30 minutes.

6. Remove the foil and bake for an additional 10 minutes until the peppers are tender.

7. Serve warm.

Nutritional Value (per serving):

- Calories: 220

- Protein: 8g

- Carbohydrates: 38g

- Fiber: 10g

- Fat: 6g

- Sodium: 250mg

5. Spinach and Chickpea Soup

Servings:4

Cooking Time: 30 minutes

Ingredients:

- ❖ 1 tablespoon olive oil

- ❖ 1 onion, chopped

- ❖ 2 garlic cloves, minced

- ❖ 1 carrot, diced

- ❖ 1 celery stalk, diced

- ❖ 4 cups low-sodium vegetable broth

- ❖ 1 can (15 oz) chickpeas, drained and rinsed

- ❖ 4 cups fresh spinach

- ❖ 1 teaspoon dried thyme

- ❖ Salt and pepper to taste

Preparation:

1. Heat olive oil in a large pot over medium heat.

2. Add the onion, garlic, carrot, and celery, sautéing until softened, about 5 minutes.

3. Add the vegetable broth, chickpeas, and thyme. Bring to a boil, then reduce heat and simmer for 15 minutes.

4. Add the spinach and cook for another 5 minutes until wilted.

5. Season with salt and pepper to taste and serve hot.

Nutritional Value (per serving):

- Calories: 150

- Protein: 6g

- Carbohydrates: 22g

- Fiber: 7g

- Fat: 4g

- Sodium: 200mg

6. Grilled Salmon with Asparagus

Servings:4

Cooking Time: 20 minutes

Ingredients:

- ❖ 4 salmon fillets (4 oz each)

- ❖ 1 bunch asparagus, trimmed

- ❖ 2 tablespoons olive oil

- ❖ 1 lemon, sliced

- ❖ Salt and pepper to taste

Preparation:

1. Preheat the grill to medium-high heat.

2. Drizzle 1 tablespoon of olive oil over the salmon fillets and season with salt and pepper.

3. Toss the asparagus with the remaining olive oil, salt, and pepper.

4. Grill the salmon fillets for about 4-5 minutes on each side until fully cooked.

5. Grill the asparagus for about 5 minutes until tender.

6. Serve the salmon fillets with grilled asparagus and lemon slices.

Nutritional Value (per serving):

- Calories: 280

- Protein: 28g

- Carbohydrates: 6g

- Fiber: 2g

- Fat: 16g

- Sodium: 90mg

7. Mediterranean Lentil Salad

Servings:4

Cooking Time: 25 minutes

Ingredients:

- 1 cup cooked lentils

- 1 cup cherry tomatoes, halved

- 1 cucumber, diced

- 1/4 cup red onion, finely chopped

- 1/4 cup feta cheese, crumbled

- 2 tablespoons olive oil

- 2 tablespoons lemon juice

- 1 teaspoon dried oregano

- Salt and pepper to taste

Preparation:

1. Cook the lentils according to package instructions and let them cool.

2. In a large bowl, combine the lentils, cherry tomatoes, cucumber, red onion, and feta cheese.

3. In a small bowl, whisk together the olive oil, lemon juice, oregano, salt, and pepper.

4. Pour the dressing over the salad and toss to combine.

5. Serve chilled or at room temperature.

Nutritional Value (per serving):

- Calories: 220

- Protein: 10g

- Carbohydrates: 25g

- Fiber: 8g

- Fat: 8g

- Sodium: 180mg

Servings:4

Cooking Time: 25 minutes

Ingredients:

- ❖ 2 chicken breasts, cubed

- ❖ 1 red bell pepper, cubed

- ❖ 1 green bell pepper, cubed

- ❖ 1 zucchini, sliced

- ❖ 1 red onion, cubed

- ❖ 2 tablespoons olive oil

- ❖ 2 tablespoons lemon juice

- ❖ 1 teaspoon dried rosemary

- ❖ Salt and pepper to taste

Preparation:

1. Preheat the grill to medium-high heat.

2. In a large bowl, combine the olive oil, lemon juice, rosemary, salt, and pepper.

3. Add the chicken and vegetables to the bowl, tossing to coat.

4. Thread the chicken and vegetables onto skewers.

5. Grill the skewers for about 10-12 minutes, turning occasionally, until the chicken is fully cooked.

6. Serve immediately.

Nutritional Value (per serving):

- Calories: 200

- Protein: 20g

- Carbohydrates: 10g

- Fiber: 3g

- Fat: 10g

- Sodium: 90mg

9. Cauliflower Rice Stir-Fry

Servings:4

Cooking Time: 20 minutes

Ingredients:

- 1 head cauliflower, grated or riced

- 1 cup mixed vegetables (carrots, peas, bell peppers)

- 1/4 cup green onions, chopped

- 2 tablespoons olive oil

- 2 tablespoons low-sodium soy sauce

- 1 teaspoon ginger, grated

- 1 garlic clove, minced

- 1 egg, beaten (optional)

Preparation:

1. Heat olive oil in a large skillet over medium heat.

2. Add the ginger and garlic, sautéing for 1 minute until fragrant.

3. Add the mixed vegetables and cook for about 5 minutes until tender.

4. Add the cauliflower rice, stirring to combine.

5. Cook for another 5 minutes until the cauliflower is tender.

6. Stir in the soy sauce and green onions.

7. If using, push the mixture to one side of the skillet and pour the beaten egg into the empty side. Scramble until fully cooked and then mix into the cauliflower rice.

8. Serve immediately.

Nutritional Value (per serving):

- Calories: 120

- Protein: 4g

- Carbohydrates: 12g

- Fiber: 5g

- Fat: 7g

- Sodium: 180mg

10. Tuna Salad with Avocado

Servings:4

Cooking Time: 15 minutes

Ingredients:

- ❖ 2 cans (5 oz each) tuna in water, drained

- ❖ 1 avocado, diced

- ❖ 1/4 cup red onion, finely chopped

- ❖ 1/4 cup celery, finely chopped

- ❖ 2 tablespoons Greek yogurt (low-fat)

- ❖ 1 tablespoon lemon juice

- ❖ Salt and pepper to taste

Preparation:

1. In a large bowl, combine the tuna, avocado, red onion, and celery.

2. In a small bowl, whisk together the Greek yogurt, lemon juice, salt, and pepper.

3. Pour the dressing over the tuna mixture and toss gently to combine.

4. Serve immediately, either on its own or with a side of whole-grain crackers.

Nutritional Value (per serving):

- Calories: 180

- Protein: 20g

- Carbohydrates: 6g

- Fiber: 4g

- Fat: 8g

- Sodium: 220mg

CHAPTER 5

DINNER RECIPES

1. Baked Lemon Herb Salmon

Servings:4

Ingredients:

- ❖ 4 salmon fillets

- ❖ 2 tablespoons olive oil

- ❖ 1 lemon (juiced and zested)

- ❖ 2 cloves garlic (minced)

- ❖ 1 teaspoon dried oregano

- ❖ 1 teaspoon dried thyme

- ❖ Salt and pepper to taste

Instructions:

1. Preheat your oven to 375°F (190°C).

2. Place salmon fillets on a baking dish lined with parchment paper.

3. In a small bowl, mix together olive oil, lemon juice, lemon zest, minced garlic, oregano, thyme, salt, and pepper.

4. Pour the mixture over the salmon fillets, making sure they are evenly coated.

5. Bake in the preheated oven for 12-15 minutes, or until salmon is cooked through and flakes easily with a fork.

6. Serve hot with your choice of steamed vegetables or a side salad.

Nutritional Values (per serving):

- **Calories: 250 kcal**

- **Carbohydrates: 2g**

- **Protein: 28g**

- **Fat: 14g**

- **Sodium: 100mg**

2. Quinoa Stuffed Bell Peppers

Servings:6

Ingredients:

- ❖ 6 bell peppers (any color)

- ❖ 1 cup quinoa, rinsed

- ❖ 2 cups vegetable broth

- ❖ 1 onion, diced

- ❖ 2 cloves garlic, minced

- ❖ 1 cup diced tomatoes

- ❖ 1 cup black beans, drained and rinsed

- ❖ 1 teaspoon cumin

- ❖ 1 teaspoon paprika

- ❖ Salt and pepper to taste

- ❖ Fresh cilantro for garnish (optional)

Instructions:

1. Preheat your oven to 375°F (190°C).
2. Cut the tops off the bell peppers and remove the seeds and membranes. Place the peppers upright in a baking dish.
3. In a saucepan, bring vegetable broth to a boil. Add quinoa, reduce heat, cover, and simmer for 15 minutes or until quinoa is cooked and liquid is absorbed.
4. In a separate skillet, heat olive oil over medium heat. Add diced onion and minced garlic, sauté until softened.
5. Add diced tomatoes, black beans, cumin, paprika, salt, and pepper to the skillet. Cook for 5 minutes, stirring occasionally.
6. Add cooked quinoa to the skillet and mix until well combined.
7. Spoon the quinoa mixture into the hollowed-out bell peppers.
8. Cover the baking dish with foil and bake for 25-30 minutes, or until the peppers are tender.
9. Garnish with fresh cilantro before serving, if desired.

Nutritional Values (per serving):

- **Calories: 220 kcal**

- **Carbohydrates: 30g**

- **Protein: 8g**

- **Fat: 7g**

- **Sodium: 150mg**

3. Ginger Turmeric Chicken Stir-Fry

Servings: 4

Ingredients:

- ❖ 1 lb chicken breast, cut into strips

- ❖ 2 tablespoons olive oil

- ❖ 2 cloves garlic, minced

- ❖ 1 tablespoon grated ginger

- ❖ 1 tablespoon turmeric powder

- ❖ 2 cups mixed vegetables (bell peppers, broccoli, carrots, snap peas)

- ❖ 2 tablespoons low-sodium soy sauce

- ❖ Salt and pepper to taste

- ❖ Sesame seeds for garnish (optional)

- ❖ Cooked brown rice for serving

Instructions:

1. Heat olive oil in a large skillet or wok over medium-high heat.

2. Add minced garlic and grated ginger to the skillet, cook for 1 minute until fragrant.

3. Add chicken strips to the skillet, season with turmeric powder, salt, and pepper. Cook until chicken is no longer pink, about 5-7 minutes.

4. Add mixed vegetables to the skillet, stir-fry for another 5 minutes or until vegetables are tender-crisp.

5. Pour low-sodium soy sauce over the chicken and vegetable mixture, toss to coat evenly.

6. Cook for an additional 2 minutes, then remove from heat.

7. Serve hot over cooked brown rice, garnish with sesame seeds if desired.

Nutritional Values (per serving):

- **Calories: 280 kcal**

- **Carbohydrates: 10g**

- **Protein: 30g**

- **Fat: 12g**

- **Sodium: 200mg**

4. Lentil and Vegetable Soup
Servings:6

Ingredients:

- ❖ 1 cup green lentils, rinsed

- ❖ 6 cups vegetable broth

- ❖ 1 onion, diced

- ❖ 2 carrots, diced

- ❖ 2 celery stalks, diced

- ❖ 2 cloves garlic, minced

- ❖ 1 teaspoon dried thyme

- ❖ 1 teaspoon dried oregano

- ❖ Salt and pepper to taste

- ❖ Fresh parsley for garnish (optional)

Instructions:

1. In a large pot, bring vegetable broth to a boil.

2. Add green lentils, diced onion, carrots, celery, minced garlic, dried thyme, dried oregano, salt, and pepper to the pot.

3. Reduce heat to low, cover, and simmer for 30-35 minutes, or until lentils and vegetables are tender.

4. Taste and adjust seasoning if necessary.

5. Serve hot, garnished with fresh parsley if desired.

Nutritional Values (per serving):

- **Calories: 180 kcal**

- **Carbohydrates: 30g**

- **Protein: 10g**

- **Fat: 2g**

- **Sodium: 200mg**

5. Grilled Lemon Herb Chicken Breast

Servings: 4

Ingredients:

- ❖ 4 boneless, skinless chicken breasts
- ❖ 2 tablespoons olive oil
- ❖ 1 lemon (juiced)
- ❖ 2 cloves garlic, minced
- ❖ 1 teaspoon dried oregano
- ❖ 1 teaspoon dried thyme
- ❖ Salt and pepper to taste

Instructions:

1. In a small bowl, whisk together olive oil, lemon juice, minced garlic, dried oregano, dried thyme, salt, and pepper.

2. Place chicken breasts in a shallow dish and pour the marinade over them. Make sure the chicken is well coated.

3. Cover and refrigerate for at least 30 minutes to marinate.

4. Preheat grill to medium-high heat.

5. Remove chicken from marinade and discard excess marinade.

6. Grill chicken breasts for 6-8 minutes per side, or until they are cooked through and no longer pink in the center.

7. Remove from grill and let rest for a few minutes before serving.

8. Serve hot with steamed vegetables or a side salad.

Nutritional Values (per serving):

- **Calories: 200 kcal**

- **Carbohydrates: 1g**

- **Protein: 30g**

- **Fat: 8g**

Sodium: 150m

6. Roasted Vegetable Quinoa Bowl

Servings: 4

Ingredients:

- ❖ 1 cup quinoa, rinsed

- ❖ 2 cups vegetable broth

- ❖ 1 sweet potato, peeled and diced

- ❖ 1 zucchini, sliced

- ❖ 1 red bell pepper, sliced

- ❖ 1 yellow bell pepper, sliced

- ❖ 1 tablespoon olive oil

- ❖ 1 teaspoon dried thyme

- ❖ 1 teaspoon dried rosemary

- ❖ Salt and pepper to taste

- ❖ Fresh parsley for garnish (optional)

Instructions:

1. Preheat your oven to 400°F (200°C).

2. In a saucepan, bring vegetable broth to a boil. Add quinoa, reduce heat, cover, and simmer for 15 minutes or until quinoa is cooked and liquid is absorbed.

3. On a large baking sheet, toss diced sweet potato, sliced zucchini, sliced red bell pepper, and sliced yellow bell pepper with olive oil, dried thyme, dried rosemary, salt, and pepper.

4. Spread the vegetables in a single layer on the baking sheet.

5. Roast in the preheated oven for 25-30 minutes, or until vegetables are tender and slightly caramelized.

6. To assemble the bowls, divide cooked quinoa among serving bowls and top with roasted vegetables.

7. Garnish with fresh parsley if desired.

Nutritional Values (per serving):

- **Calories: 230 kcal**

- **Carbohydrates: 30g**

- **Protein: 8g**

- **Fat: 10g**

- **Sodium: 100mg**

7. Turkey and Vegetable Skillet

Servings:4

Ingredients:

- ❖ 1 lb ground turkey

- ❖ 2 tablespoons olive oil

- ❖ 1 onion, diced

- ❖ 2 cloves garlic, minced

- ❖ 2 cups mixed vegetables (bell peppers, broccoli, carrots, snap peas)

- ❖ 1 teaspoon dried basil

- ❖ 1 teaspoon dried oregano

- ❖ Salt and pepper to taste

Instructions:

1. Heat olive oil in a large skillet over medium heat.

2. Add diced onion and minced garlic to the skillet, cook until softened.

3. Add ground turkey to the skillet, breaking it up with a spatula. Cook until turkey is browned and cooked through.

4. Add mixed vegetables to the skillet, season with dried basil, dried oregano, salt, and pepper. Cook for 5-7 minutes, or until vegetables are tender-crisp.

5. Taste and adjust seasoning if necessary.

6. Serve hot.

   Nutritional Values (per serving):

- **Calories: 240 kcal**

- **Carbohydrates: 10g**

- **Protein: 25g**

- **Fat: 12g**

- **Sodium: 180mg**

Servings:4

Ingredients:

- ❖ 1 lb shrimp, peeled and deveined

- ❖ 4 medium zucchini

- ❖ 2 tablespoons olive oil

- ❖ 4 cloves garlic, minced

- ❖ 1 lemon (juiced and zested)

- ❖ Salt and pepper to taste

- ❖ Fresh parsley for garnish (optional)

Instructions:

1. Using a spiralizer, spiralize the zucchini into noodles. Set aside.

2. Heat olive oil in a large skillet over medium heat.

3. Add minced garlic to the skillet, cook until fragrant.

4. Add shrimp to the skillet, season with salt, pepper, lemon juice, and lemon zest. Cook until shrimp is pink and cooked through.

5. Remove shrimp from the skillet and set aside.

6. In the same skillet, add zucchini noodles. Cook for 2-3 minutes, or until noodles are just tender.

7. Return cooked shrimp to the skillet and toss to combine with the zucchini noodles.

8. Serve hot, garnished with fresh parsley if desired.

Nutritional Values (per serving):

- **Calories: 180 kcal**

- **Carbohydrates: 8g**

- **Protein: 25g**

- **Fat: 6g**

- **Sodium: 200mg**

9. Baked Herb Chicken with Roasted Vegetables

Servings: 4

Ingredients:

- ❖ 4 boneless, skinless chicken breasts

- ❖ 2 tablespoons olive oil

- ❖ 1 teaspoon dried basil

- ❖ 1 teaspoon dried thyme

- ❖ 1 teaspoon dried rosemary

- ❖ 2 cups mixed vegetables (bell peppers, broccoli, carrots, snap peas)

- ❖ Salt and pepper to taste

Instructions:

1. Preheat your oven to 375°F (190°C).

2. Place chicken breasts in a baking dish.

3. In a small bowl, mix together olive oil, dried basil, dried thyme, dried rosemary, salt, and pepper.

4. Pour the herb mixture over the chicken breasts, making sure they are evenly coated.

5. Arrange mixed vegetables around the chicken breasts in the baking dish.

6. Bake in the preheated oven for 25-30 minutes, or until chicken is cooked through and vegetables are tender.

7. Serve hot.

Nutritional Values (per serving):

- **Calories: 230 kcal**

- **Carbohydrates: 10g**

- **Protein: 30g**

- **Fat: 8g**

- **Sodium: 150mg**

10. Spinach and Mushroom Omelette

Servings:2

Ingredients:

- ❖ 4 eggs

- ❖ 1 cup fresh spinach leaves

- ❖ 1/2 cup sliced mushrooms

- ❖ 1/4 cup diced onion

- ❖ 2 tablespoons olive oil

- ❖ Salt and pepper to taste

Instructions:

1. In a bowl, beat eggs until well mixed. Season with salt and pepper.

2. Heat olive oil in a non-stick skillet over medium heat.

3. Add diced onion and sliced mushrooms to the skillet, cook until softened.

4. Add fresh spinach leaves to the skillet, cook until wilted.

5. Pour beaten eggs over the vegetables in the skillet.

6. Cook until the edges of the omelette start to set,
    then gently lift the edges with a spatula and tilt the
    skillet to let the uncooked eggs flow to the bottom.

7. Once the omelette is mostly set, fold it in half and
    cook for another minute or until cooked through.

8. Slide the omelette onto a plate and serve hot.

Nutritional Values (per serving):

- Calories: 180 kcal

- Carbohydrates: 5g

- Protein: 12g

- Fat: 12g

- Sodium: 150mg

CONCLUSION

In conclusion, this colitis diet cookbook for seniors over 50 offers a diverse range of delicious and nutritious recipes tailored to support digestive health while providing essential nutrients for overall well-being. By focusing on natural, low-sugar, low-carb, low-sodium, and low-fat ingredients, these recipes are gentle on the digestive system, making them ideal for individuals managing colitis, heart disease, and kidney issues.

Through careful selection of ingredients and detailed step-by-step instructions, this cookbook empowers seniors to take control of their diet and embrace flavorful meals that promote healing and alleviate symptoms associated with colitis. From comforting soups and hearty stews to light salads and protein-packed entrees, there is something for every taste preference and dietary need.

But beyond the culinary aspect, adopting this colitis-friendly diet offers seniors a pathway to improved quality of life. By nourishing the body with wholesome, nutrient-dense foods, individuals may experience reduced inflammation, better digestion, increased energy levels, and enhanced overall health. Moreover, embracing this diet can foster a sense of empowerment and control over one's health journey, instilling confidence and peace of mind.

As you embark on this culinary adventure, remember that each recipe is not just a meal but a step towards a healthier, more vibrant life. Let the flavors tantalize your taste buds, the nourishment invigorate your body, and the joy of cooking bring fulfillment to your soul. Embrace this journey with enthusiasm and determination, knowing that every bite you take is a testament to your commitment to self-care and well-being. Your health is your greatest asset—cherish it, nurture it, and let these recipes guide you towards a brighter, healthier future.

www.ingramcontent.com/pod-product-compliance
Lightning Source LLC
Chambersburg PA
CBHW081557250726
48653CB00009B/3468